# Hospital Stay - 101

I0476301

## A safety handbook
## for
## healthcare consumers

Contributors/Critiques:

Susan Andazola, RN, BSN
Minnie Magbitang, RN, BSN

Editor:

Alexandra Besket

Cover Design & Cover Photography:

Lexi T. Williams

ISBN 9781515205630

For Dr. Williams Speaking Engagements
Email: drpvwilliams@gmail.com

Website: www.drpvw.vpweb.com
facebook.com/HealthAwarenessAdvocates

# Content

# Acknowledgment

My life has been affected by many individuals, especially those who I have had the opportunity to provide medical care. As a caregiver, I experienced the challenges people face when they needed to have their health restored, and I feel that they can be more a part of that process than they think. It is that fact which inspired me to write this handbook.

The title has been seared in my mind for some time because I wanted it to be very simple, easy to read and understand. I wanted it to cover basic things which one should consider when there is an occasion to be hospitalized.

I owe a debt of gratitude to my husband and two  beautiful children for being among my biggest fans. I love you all unconditionally. I would also like to thank my close friends and church family for their support, friendship, and love.

To Patrick Peters, Founder of Senior B2B Networking, which provides Professional Services to the Senior Communities, thank you for the opportunity to speak on this subject at the Open Forums for your membership.

Finally, I am very grateful for two of my nursing friends and colleagues: Susan Andazola RN, BSN., Minnie Magbitang RN, BSN., who read, critiqued, and contributed to this handbook, as well as Alexandra Besket for her editing skills.

## About The Author

Dr. Paula V. Williams is a Registered Nurse who has more than twenty-eight years of experience in providing patient care, management, and leadership in the hospital setting.

She is a University Adjunct Nursing Professor, and is trained in many disciplines of the nursing profession. She has been published, and was the recipient of the CAPPS Award when she graduated with her Associate Nursing Degree.

She was inducted into the Sigma Theta Tau International Honor Society of Nursing, as the top BSN graduate (Bachelor of Science in Nursing). She holds an MSN (Masters of Science in Nursing) degree, a MBA/HCM (Masters Business Administration in Health Care

Management), and a PhD in Public Health, graduating with high honors and invited into the Golden Key International Honour Society.

She was a proud recipient of Dignity Health's, 2014 Humankindness Award.

## Purpose

The purpose of this handbook is to educate the public with some basic information they should know when being admitted into the hospital/medical center for treatment.

The mandate of hospitals and their medical personnel is to provide the best care possible for the benefit of restoring the patient to optimum health. On becoming a knowledgeable healthcare consumer, you will be armed to be proactive and engaged in your medical treatment and recovery.

Thank you for the privilege to share this important information.

Dr. Williams can be reached by email at: drpvwilliams@gmail.com

# Hospital Stay - 101

YOUR LIFE, ONE LIFE – PROTECT IT! You can help to protect yourself from medical harm. Admission to the hospital as a patient can expose you to the possibility of medical errors. Remember, humans make mistakes.

## Personal Advocate

It is encouraged to have a trusted advocate with you. Your advocate could be a family member, or close friend who will be able to ask questions and seek answers on your behalf during your stay in the hospital.

Inform the staff with the name(s) of your designated advocate(s). This person will not be responsible for signing legal documents on your behalf, unless outlined in your Health Care Directive.

## Nurse Advocate

Your registered nurse (RN) is your professional advocate who will be executing the doctors' orders to treat your illness or disease.

## What To Bring

Bring a journal with you to write things down. The staff tends to be more attentive, conscientious, and cautious if you, your loved one, or advocate displays an interest in what they are doing and the manner in which they are caring for you.

On your visit to the hospital, have your driver's license, or a form of governmental identification and insurance information ready to present for registration. It is important to give a complete and accurate account of the nature of your illness, including the time of the onset of your symptoms.

If you have chronic conditions, such as high blood pressure, diabetes, kidney disease, or heart issues, inform the RN and your doctor. It is a good idea to print and have your health history with you, including the last date you had any X-rays, EKGs, Scans, or Ultrasounds completed. This will avoid the omission of any important information relating to your care.

If you are taking medications, make sure you bring the medications, or bring your complete up-to-date medication list. The list should include the name of the medications, the correct dosage, how often they are taken, the last date and time you took any medication(s). This is important for the doctor to know, so that while you are in the hospital, he or she can make the decision to continue or discontinue any of your medications, where appropriate, for your best benefit.

It would help to have a list of the names of your current doctors and their specialties. This will assist the hospital doctors in coordinating your care. Some doctors are specialists and may be contracted with the hospital. Ask if the doctor(s) attending to you, or reading your X-rays, Scans, or Ultrasounds are covered under your health insurance. If they are not, you may request to have a doctor who accepts your insurance. This will avoid a high out-of-pocket hospital bill after your recovery.

Should you have an allergy to any medications, make sure that an allergy alert armband is placed on your wrist indicating that you have an allergy.

Other armbands to expect, where applicable, are: Blood Transfusion, Safety/Fall Risk, Nothing by Mouth, Avoidance of an arm that should not be used for blood pressure, blood work, IV (intravenous) fluids, etc.

Finally, if you have a Healthcare Directive, it is a good idea to bring it with you. If you do not already have one, you may follow up with a hospital representative to create one. This will serve to carry out your wishes for medical treatment if you are unable to communicate, or provide consent.

### Be Involved

Know your vital signs i.e. temperature, heart rate, blood pressure, respirations and oxygenation. Ask the staff member what your readings are and compare the readings each time the staff member takes your vital signs. You should be aware if the readings are abnormal. The nurse must intervene, treat, and monitor you to make sure you return to stability.

For example, if you have a history of high blood pressure, be sure to pay close attention to your blood pressure readings. If the reading is higher than what you know to be your normal, it needs to be addressed by your nurse; if your blood pressure is too low, make sure you have a discussion with your nurse about it as well, and avoid taking any medication(s) that could further lower your blood pressure.

## Staff Identification

Hold everyone accountable for their role in your care. When the hospital staff introduces him or herself, check and ensure that they are wearing a visible name badge. Know their names, titles, and roles; better yet, write their names down and familiarize yourself with them. Some hospitals require their staff to wear color-coded uniforms which identify their role/job expertise. Ask your nurse to explain the different roles and their designated colors where applicable.

## Doctors in your care

Familiarize yourself with the doctors caring for you, including their name(s) and specialties. Write their names down. Ask each doctor involved about your progress and his or her plan for you. Write down your requests, questions, or concerns and have a candid discussion with your doctors when they come in to see you.

This is a good time to have any requests filled. Remember that the doctor(s) involved in your care may not be available after hours. Doctors "On Call" are in place to address any after hour needs (if your regular doctor(s) are off duty). Be aware that the doctor on call may hesitate to fulfill non-emergent requests due to lack of familiarity with you and your plan of care.

## Role of the CNA/PCT

Some units may have CNAs [Certified Nursing Assistant(s), or PCTs (Patient Care Technician(s)]. Their role is to assist the RN to care for you. They are responsible for: taking your vital signs, filling your water pitcher, providing nourishment as your diet permits, assisting with your hygiene, changing your bed linen, provide pillow cases, blankets, towels, washcloths, emptying catheters, turning and repositioning you, as necessary, (at least every two hours), assisting you to the restroom (if safe to do so), removing excess garbage and dirty laundry from your room etc.

## Chain of Command

Your RN ensures that all your needs are met. In every hospital, or facility, there is a chain of command. There may be an occasion where you may not be pleased with those caring for you (perhaps a personality conflict, or a feeling that the staff is not performing to your comfort); ask for the Charge Nurse or Unit Manager, and request a staffing change.

It is important to have a feeling of comfort, confidence and trust in your caregivers. Request, and write in your journal, the telephone extensions of the Charge Nurse, Manager, or Unit

Director. Be sure to let them know your concerns or any positive feedback regarding those caring for you; it will be appreciated.

## Safety

SAFETY is a hospital priority. Wearing non-skid slippers (may be provided) is highly recommended to help avoid falls. Call for assistance if you do not feel safe to get out of your bed or chair. Where necessary, use the approved device such as cane, crutches, or walker to assist you when walking. Make sure you are comfortable with the degree of lighting in your room at nights, especially if you are up walking independently.

## Handwashing

Observe and ensure that all staff washes their hands when they enter your room. This is a hospital expectation and the best line of defense to prevent infections. Always wash your hands as well, and also encourage your visitors to wash their hands when they enter your room.

## Calling for Assistance

Your call bell or call light should be within your reach, and accessible at all times. When you are in the bathroom and need assistance, alert the staff by using the emergency call bell or call light and wait. Do not attempt to return to your bed or chair unaccompanied.

## Repositioning in bed

If you are able, turn & reposition yourself at least every one to two hours to prevent the breakdown of your skin due to prolonged pressure in one position. If you are unable to do so independently, make sure that the staff changes your position for the same reason.

## Treatment Plan

You are to receive an explanation of your treatment plan and what you can expect during your hospital stay. This plan should be updated with you on a daily basis, as you progress towards recovery, or even if your recovery is slowed. Make sure that the treatment plan and expectations are discussed with your nurses each shift. Ask questions if you are uncertain, or if you do not understand the information.

Inquire about the doctor(s) orders, including doctors consulted to be a part of your care. Know your approved diet, Activity, IV fluids, IV medications, Tests: Blood work, X-rays, Scans, Ultrasounds, or any Special Precautions etc.

## Medications

When you are given any medications, know the name, purpose of the drug(s), and any side-effects. Note the time medications are being administered and ask how often you can expect to receive them. Having this knowledge will help you and your nurse keep the medication administration within the appropriate time frame. This will avoid you receiving the medication too early, too late, missing a dose, or receiving a duplicate dose.

If it is your desire to continue your home medication regiment, inform your nurse. He or she will communicate your desire to the hospital's pharmacist to ensure that you continue receiving your medications at the time to which you are accustomed. Remember the general rule: **Right** person, **Right** medication, **Right** dose, **Right** route and **Right** time.

The nurse must tell you what medication is being given, the dose, the reason for the administration and any possible side-effects. Do not swallow or allow any medication into your IV, applied to your skin, given rectally, by inhalation, or injection unless you know what is being given and the reason. If you must, ask to see the medication in its package to verify.

## Intravenous Access (I.V.)

If you are required to have I.V. access, and you know from past experience that accessing your vein has been challenging, make a request for the staff member with the greatest expertise at starting IVs to initiate it. This may help to minimize multiple needle-sticks.

A functioning IV site is to be used for three to four days (based on hospital policy), ask your RN how long you can expect to have it in.

After three or four days it needs to be removed and a new IV site established. The IV site and dressing should always be flat, clean, dry, and well-secured. If the site becomes red,  swollen, painful, bleeds, or begins to leak fluids, notify your nurse immediately.  For these reasons, the site may need to be changed before the three to four day expiration.

### Port or Pacemaker

Should you have a port, pacemaker, or internal defibrillator, it is important to have the appliance's identification card with you.

The information on the card is of great importance to your nursing and medical staff as it plays an intricate part in your care.

## Blood Samples

You may need to give blood samples for testing. Be sure to ask what tests are being done, and ask for the results so that you can also monitor if the results show an improvement or worsening of your condition. Ask for an explanation of any abnormal blood work results. This will help you to stay current on your progress. If the results are abnormal, find out from your RN or doctor what plans can be expected to address them.

Know what time you can expect your blood sample to be obtained, (some are obtained in relation to certain medications). Knowing when your blood sample will be taken, will alert you should the phlebotomist (the person who obtains blood samples) comes in unexpectedly to obtain your blood specimen.

At this point, before you are stuck with a needle, ask why the specimen is needed. If you are anticipating the collection of a routine blood specimen, and obtaining the current sample is, for example, one or two hours away from the routine collection time, ask the phlebotomist to check with your nurse. Your nurse is able to determine if the collection of all the blood samples required can be done in a single attempt. You would have saved yourself from an extra needlestick. Again, ask for the results, this includes blood sugar checks, if you are a person with diabetes. Know what other tests are ordered and ask for the results for comparison. Be engaged and monitor your progress.

## Informed Consent(s)

Be fully informed regarding your surgery or procedure. Education must precede all consent(s); DO NOT sign a consent(s), unless you have received an explanation from a medical professional knowledgeable about, and directly involved in your surgery or procedure. Make sure all your questions and concerns are addressed, and you have a full understanding. Remember your personal advocate can also ask questions on your behalf.

## Medical Terminologies

Should the staff use medical terminologies you do not understand, let them know, and ask for a simple explanation. Seek other resources to assist you in being an informed patient, and healthcare consumer. There are multiple websites and books that will define and help you understand medical terminologies

## Do Not Wait

If you have an emergency, do not hesitate to do what you need to do to get immediate attention.  If you are not "feeling right", such as increased shortness of breath, lightheadedness or feeling faint, call your nurse for immediate attention. If there is a delay in the staff responding to you, dial "0" for the hospital operator; inform the operator of your room number and that you need immediate assistance.

## DVT – Deep Vein Thrombosis

Your activity level may be reduced while you are in the hospital and diminished blood circulation to your lower legs can cause the pooling of blood causing clot formation.

Medications called anticoagulants may be ordered for you by the doctor to help prevent blood clots (DVT – deep vein thrombosis).

Displacement of a blood clot(s) could result in what is known as pulmonary embolism (release of the blood clot into the blood stream and lodging in the lungs), which can be life-threatening.

There are devices called SCD (sequential compression device) that may be placed on your lower legs to assist with circulation when you are in bed. While in bed, pump and rotate your ankles, exercise your legs to promote circulation.

## Expectations After Surgery

After surgery, remember to deep breathe and cough to exercise your lungs. Make sure, where appropriate and ordered by your surgeon, that the staff assists you to get up out of bed. This will help your digestive system return to normal. Make sure you receive stool softeners (where appropriate) to avoid constipation. Your nurse will be assessing you for bowel sounds, the expulsion of digestive gas, and bowel movements, which are indicative of your digestive system returning to normal.

## Surgical Dressing

Your surgical dressing should be clean, dry, and intact. The nurse will monitor your surgical site for any drainage or developing infection. If your dressing needs to be changed, it should be done under sterile conditions. This will decrease risk of an infection to your incision.

## Drainage Collection Devices

Drainage collection devices should be monitored and emptied, or changed before they become full. Drain(s) to your wounds may be connected to suction, most commonly a compressed suction (which will help to remove excess drainage from the wound and promote healing). To be effective, drain(s) should be compressed (per the surgeon's order); there are situations where the drains may need to be decompressed. The RN should explain the reasons to you. Check with your nurse to make sure that all equipment related to your care is functioning.

## Changing Shift

Most shift changes are at 6 or 7 a.m./p.m. Plan ahead. An hour or two before the shift changes, plan to address all your needs with your RN such as pain, nausea, bathroom trips, fresh water, towels etc.

Capitalize on the attention of the staff to address your needs when they are in your room. Once the staff leaves your room, they may be attending to other patients and unable to respond to you in a timely fashion.

## Discharge

Inquire regarding when you can expect to be discharged, so that you can begin to make post-hospitalization plans. The Case Manager or Social Worker will be able to assist if you have additional discharge needs.

At discharge you should receive clear written and verbal instructions on your post-hospitalization care, including a list of your current medications, prescriptions, follow-up doctors' appointments, and how to take care of yourself when you return home.

## Goal

Your goal is to leave the hospital safely, in the shortest amount of time, and be on the road to recovery.

## Speak-Up, Ask Questions, Get Answers

SPEAK-UP, continue to educate yourself, and be an involved patient to protect yourself from avoidable mistakes.

## PATIENT RIGHTS & RESPONSIBILITIES

Do ask for, and read a copy of the hospital's *Patient Rights & Responsibilities. It will inform you about your rights and your responsibilities as a patient/healthcare consumer.

Note: You can report any patient safety issues or concern about quality to the hospital's safety officer and/or The Joint Commission.

Contact number for The Commission is:

1-800-994-6610, Fax: 630-792-5636
E-mail: complaint@jointcommission.org
Mail: Office of Quality Monitoring
The Joint Commission
One Renaissance Boulevard
Oakbrook Terrace, Illinois 60181

## *What Is the Patient Bill of Rights?

Medical facilities have always had regulations covering patient information and standard practices, but the Health Insurance Portability and Accountability Act (HIPAA) of 1996, The Consumer Bill of Rights and Responsibilities of 1998 and the patient Safety Act of 2005, are among the legislative acts and reports that make up a legally binding Patient Bill of Rights.

Many states have codified Patient rights, and special rights exist for conditions like mental illness and hospice patients.

## Informed Consent

Patients have the right to the information necessary to make decisions about their health care that is provided in their primary language in ways they can understand.

## Choice

Patients have the right and the responsibility to choose health care providers they trust and who they believe are best able to treat them successfully.

## Access

Individuals deserve immediate access to emergency medical care when needed-- without waiting for authorizations--if their health is in serious danger or they are suffering from a serious injury.

## Active Participation

Patients have the right to know options and the responsibility to participate in decisions regarding their healthcare, or to authorize a representative to make decisions for them.

## Respect

Patients have the right to respect and consideration, and should never suffer from discrimination based on differences by healthcare professionals or healthcare plan representatives.

## Confidentiality

Patients have the right to consult privately with their healthcare providers, to see and discuss their personal medical records and to request changes to those records: privacy protocols are specifically listed in HIPAA.

## Complaints

Patients must have access to policy outlining a procedure that guarantees a timely, confidential and fair review of any complaints they may have concerning care, facilities and personnel, or their healthcare insurer.

## Sample Journal

**Date :**

**Doctors :**

**Nurse:**

**CNA or PCT:**

**Care plan:**

**Tests done:**

**Results:**

**Antibiotic(s):**

**Questions:**

# Comments

"A must have for any patient or family navigating the healthcare systems of America. Information is the key to safety and easing fears - this handbook provides that information in an easy to understand manner."

Kevin Meek, RN, MHI
Chief Nursing Officer
Dignity Health-Arizona General Hospital


"Dr. Paula Williams is a wonderful dedicated professional who cares deeply for her patients and community. I am delighted and honored to have been able to review this handbook for her, and wish that every Patient and family (of the Patient)admitted to hospital has ample opportunity to review the contents, and use the tools provided to empower themselves in the delivery of healthcare and their healthcare choices. This handbook will change lives!"

Yagnesh B. Patel, MD
Internal Medicine/Hospitalist
Chief of Staff
Chandler Regional and
Mercy Gilbert Medical Centers, AZ

"Sooner or later we or our loved ones are going to be in a hospital as patients. Whether the hospital stay is for a routine care, or a sudden serious emergency, there are things that we need to know in order to have a healthy stay".

"Dr. Williams has provided an inside information, on healthy hospital stays, that every person needs. The Handbook is well written and provides all the pertinent information that non-health professionals can understand. This is a must-have document for everyone."

Peter Okrah, Ph.D.
Electrical Engineer
Phoenix, AZ.


"Important information for every patient to have. A must have for inpatient care."

Shaneeta Johnson MD FACS, FICS
Minimally Invasive and Bariatric Surgeon
Atlanta, GA.

Your Life, One Life, - Protect it!